THE DIABETIC COOKBOOK AND MEAL PLAN FOR THE NEWLY DIAGNOSED

Master Diabetes Meals from Day One with Flavorful Recipes & a 4-Week Plan

T. John

COPYRIGHT PAGE

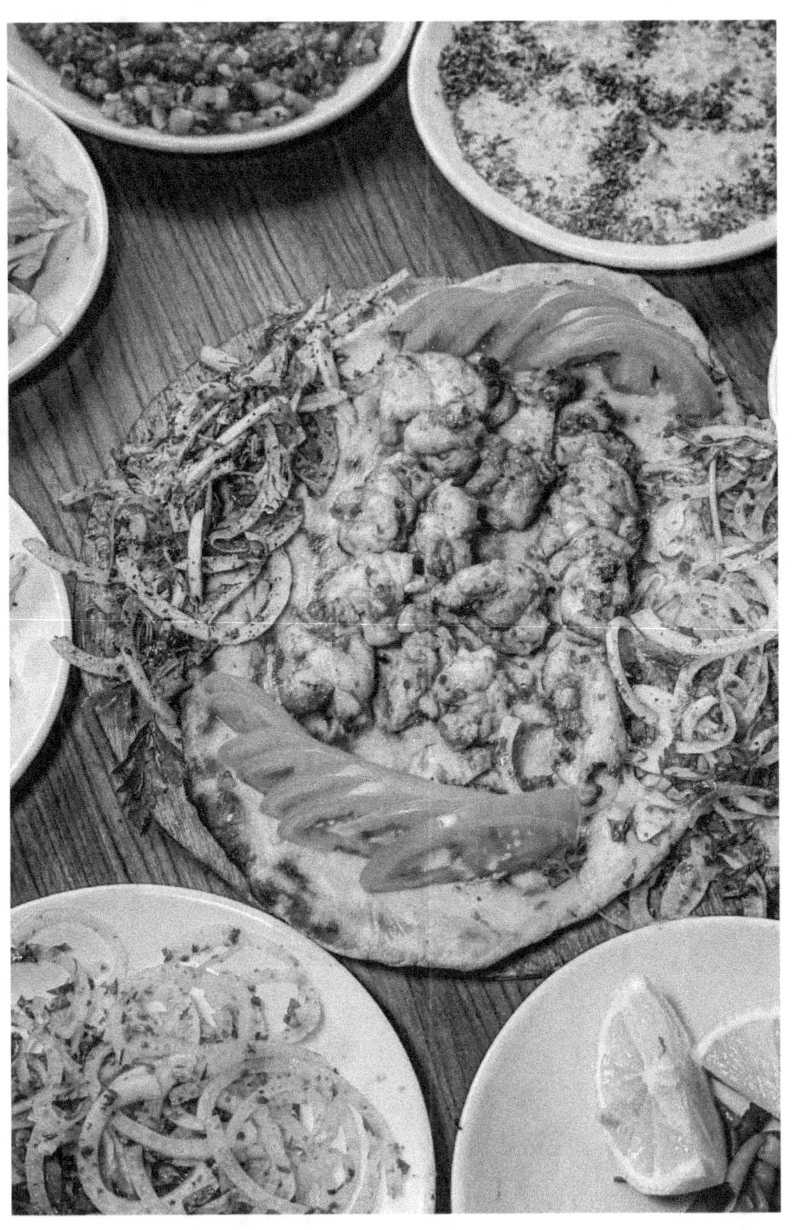

TABLE OF CONTENTS

Chapter 5: Snacks and Appetizers 82

INTRODUCTION

Imagine your body as a bustling city, humming with activity. Glucose, the fuel for this metropolis, arrives from the food you eat, delivered by couriers called insulin. In diabetes, though, this system gets a bit wonky. Either the couriers are scarce (type 1) or the city gates resist their entry (type 2). The sugar then hangs around, causing chaos – that's what we call high blood sugar.

But here's the good news: you're not just a bystander in this urban drama. The food you choose becomes your secret weapon, influencing how smoothly your city runs. Think of it as strategic urban planning for your body!

Let's build a foundation of smart choices:

- **Whole grains over refined carbs**: Swap white bread for brown rice, opt for quinoa over couscous. These complex carbs release sugar slowly, preventing energy spikes and crashes.

- **Colorful friends, plentiful greens**: Load your plate with veggies like broccoli and peppers, and fruits like berries and apples. They're packed with vitamins, minerals, and fiber, which help regulate blood sugar and keep you feeling full.

- **Lean protein for steady energy**: Chicken, fish, lentils, and beans are your powerhouses. They provide sustained energy without triggering blood sugar fluctuations.

- **Healthy fats, the unsung heroes**: Olive oil, avocado, and nuts are your allies. They keep you satiated, improve insulin sensitivity, and add flavor to your meals.

Remember, portion control is key: Think of your plate as a pie chart. Fill half with non-starchy veggies, a quarter with whole grains, and the remaining quarter with protein. This "smart plate" approach ensures balanced fuel distribution for your city.

Beyond the plate, consider these:

- **Timing matters**: Spread your meals and snacks evenly throughout the day to avoid blood sugar rollercoasters.
- **Hydration is crucial**: Water helps flush out excess sugar and keeps your body functioning optimally.
- **Mindful eating, a powerful tool**: Savor your food, chew slowly, and pay attention to hunger and satiety cues. This prevents overeating and promotes healthy choices.

The journey with diabetes isn't a solo trek. Seek support from a healthcare team and fellow warriors. With the right knowledge, mindful choices, and a touch of culinary creativity, you can transform your diet into a powerful tool for managing diabetes and living a vibrant, fulfilling life. Remember, you're the architect of your internal city – build it with wisdom, nourish it with care, and watch it thrive!

Chapter 1: 30-Day Meal Plan

Week 1:

Day 1:

- Breakfast: Avocado and Spinach Omelette
- Lunch: Grilled Chicken Salad with Balsamic Vinaigrette
- Dinner: Baked Cod with Lemon and Herbs
- Snack: Guacamole with Veggie Sticks
- Dessert: Berry and Yogurt Popsicles

Day 2:

- Breakfast: Greek Yogurt Parfait with Berries
- Lunch: Quinoa and Black Bean Stuffed Peppers
- Dinner: Cauliflower Rice and Chicken Curry
- Snack: Greek Yogurt and Berry Parfait
- Dessert: Dark Chocolate-Dipped Strawberries

Day 3:

- Breakfast: Quinoa Breakfast Bowl
- Lunch: Salmon and Asparagus Foil Pack

- Dinner: Beef and Vegetable Skewers
- Snack: Hummus and Whole Grain Crackers
- Dessert: Baked Apple with Cinnamon

Day 4:

- Breakfast: Whole Grain Pancakes with Sugar-Free Syrup
- Lunch: Turkey and Vegetable Stir-Fry
- Dinner: Stuffed Bell Peppers with Ground Turkey
- Snack: Cheese and Grape Skewers
- Dessert: Greek Yogurt and Honey Frozen Bites

Day 5:

- Breakfast: Vegetable and Egg Breakfast Burrito
- Lunch: Lentil Soup with Vegetables
- Dinner: Grilled Veggie and Quinoa Stuffed Portobello Mushrooms
- Snack: Roasted Chickpeas with Paprika
- Dessert: Sugar-Free Chocolate Avocado Mousse

Day 6:

- Breakfast: Chia Seed Pudding with Almonds

- Lunch: Caprese Salad with Chicken

- Dinner: Zoodle (Zucchini Noodle) Lasagna

- Snack: Cucumber and Tomato Salsa

- Dessert: Almond Flour Banana Bread

Day 7:

- Breakfast: Breakfast Casserole with Turkey Sausage

- Lunch: Whole Grain Wrap with Hummus and Vegetables

- Dinner: Lemon Garlic Roast Chicken

- Snack: Apple Slices with Almond Butter

- Dessert: Lemon Sorbet with Fresh Mint

Week 2:

Day 8:

- Breakfast: Zucchini and Feta Muffins

- Lunch: Shrimp and Quinoa Bowl

- Dinner: Spaghetti Squash with Turkey Meatballs

- Snack: Edamame with Sea Salt

- Dessert: Pumpkin Pie Chia Pudding

Day 9:

- Breakfast: Smoked Salmon and Cream Cheese Bagel
- Lunch: Chickpea and Spinach Salad
- Dinner: Teriyaki Salmon with Broccoli
- Snack: Caprese Kabobs with Balsamic Glaze
- Dessert: Coconut and Berry Parfait

Day 10:

- Breakfast: Oatmeal with Walnuts and Berries
- Lunch: Turkey and Avocado Wrap
- Dinner: Sweet Potato and Black Bean Chili
- Snack: Trail Mix with Nuts and Dried Fruit
- Dessert: Walnut and Date Energy Bites

Day 11:

- Breakfast: Cottage Cheese and Pineapple Bowl
- Lunch: Vegetable and Tofu Stir-Fry
- Dinner: Ratatouille with Chickpeas
- Snack: Veggie Spring Rolls with Peanut Sauce
- Dessert: Raspberry and Almond Tart

Day 12:

- Breakfast: Sweet Potato Hash with Poached Eggs
- Lunch: Mediterranean Quinoa Salad
- Dinner: Pesto Zucchini Noodles with Cherry Tomatoes
- Snack: Cottage Cheese and Pineapple Skewers
- Dessert: Chia Seed and Mixed Berry Jam

Day 13:

- Breakfast: Green Smoothie Bowl
- Lunch: Spinach and Feta Turkey Burger
- Dinner: Turkey and Vegetable Lettuce Wraps
- Snack: Stuffed Mushrooms with Spinach and Feta
- Dessert: Chocolate Zucchini Brownies

Day 14:

- Breakfast: Turkey and Vegetable Breakfast Wrap
- Lunch: Chicken Caesar Salad with Whole Grain Croutons
- Dinner: BBQ Chicken and Vegetable Skewers
- Snack: Avocado and Tomato Bruschetta
- Dessert: Mango and Coconut Frozen Yogurt

Week 3:

Day 15:

- Breakfast: Almond Butter and Banana Toast
- Lunch: Eggplant and Tomato Stack
- Dinner: Creamy Mushroom and Spinach Risotto
- Snack: Stuffed Mushrooms with Spinach and Feta
- Dessert: Peanut Butter and Banana Ice Cream

Day 16:

- Breakfast: Grilled Chicken Salad with Balsamic Vinaigrette
- Lunch: Quinoa and Black Bean Stuffed Peppers
- Dinner: Baked Cod with Lemon and Herbs
- Snack: Guacamole with Veggie Sticks
- Dessert: Berry and Yogurt Popsicles

Day 17:

- Breakfast: Greek Yogurt Parfait with Berries
- Lunch: Salmon and Asparagus Foil Pack
- Dinner: Cauliflower Rice and Chicken Curry
- Snack: Greek Yogurt and Berry Parfait
- Dessert: Dark Chocolate-Dipped Strawberries

Day 18:

- Breakfast: Quinoa Breakfast Bowl
- Lunch: Turkey and Vegetable Stir-Fry
- Dinner: Stuffed Bell Peppers with Ground Turkey
- Snack: Hummus and Whole Grain Crackers
- Dessert: Baked Apple with Cinnamon

Day 19:

- Breakfast: Whole Grain Pancakes with Sugar-Free Syrup
- Lunch: Lentil Soup with Vegetables
- Dinner: Grilled Veggie and Quinoa Stuffed Portobello Mushrooms
- Snack: Cheese and Grape Skewers
- Dessert: Greek Yogurt and Honey Frozen Bites

Day 20:

- Breakfast: Vegetable and Egg Breakfast Burrito
- Lunch: Caprese Salad with Chicken
- Dinner: Zoodle (Zucchini Noodle) Lasagna
- Snack: Roasted Chickpeas with Paprika
- Dessert: Almond Flour Banana Bread

Day 21:

- Breakfast: Chia Seed Pudding with Almonds
- Lunch: Whole Grain Wrap with Hummus and Vegetables
- Dinner: Lemon Garlic Roast Chicken
- Snack: Apple Slices with Almond Butter
- Dessert: Lemon Sorbet with Fresh Mint

Week 4:

Day 22:

- Breakfast: Zucchini and Feta Muffins
- Lunch: Shrimp and Quinoa Bowl
- Dinner: Spaghetti Squash with Turkey Meatballs
- Snack: Edamame with Sea Salt
- Dessert: Pumpkin Pie Chia Pudding

Day 23:

- Breakfast: Smoked Salmon and Cream Cheese Bagel
- Lunch: Chickpea and Spinach Salad
- Dinner: Teriyaki Salmon with Broccoli
- Snack: Caprese Kabobs with Balsamic Glaze
- Dessert: Coconut and Berry Parfait

Day 24:

- Breakfast: Oatmeal with Walnuts and Berries
- Lunch: Turkey and Avocado Wrap
- Dinner: Sweet Potato and Black Bean Chili
- Snack: Trail Mix with Nuts and Dried Fruit
- Dessert: Walnut and Date Energy Bites

Day 25:

- Breakfast: Cottage Cheese and Pineapple Bowl
- Lunch: Vegetable and Tofu Stir-Fry
- Dinner: Ratatouille with Chickpeas
- Snack: Veggie Spring Rolls with Peanut Sauce
- Dessert: Raspberry and Almond Tart

Day 26:

- Breakfast: Sweet Potato Hash with Poached Eggs
- Lunch: Mediterranean Quinoa Salad
- Dinner: Pesto Zucchini Noodles with Cherry Tomatoes
- Snack: Cottage Cheese and Pineapple Skewers
- Dessert: Chia Seed and Mixed Berry Jam

Day 27:

- Breakfast: Green Smoothie Bowl
- Lunch: Spinach and Feta Turkey Burger
- Dinner: Turkey and Vegetable Lettuce Wraps
- Snack: Stuffed Mushrooms with Spinach and Feta
- Dessert: Chocolate Zucchini Brownies

Day 28:

- Breakfast: Turkey and Vegetable Breakfast Wrap
- Lunch: Chicken Caesar Salad with Whole Grain Croutons
- Dinner: BBQ Chicken and Vegetable Skewers
- Snack: Avocado and Tomato Bruschetta
- Dessert: Mango and Coconut Frozen Yogurt

Day 29:

- Breakfast: Almond Butter and Banana Toast
- Lunch: Eggplant and Tomato Stack
- Dinner: Creamy Mushroom and Spinach Risotto
- Snack: Stuffed Mushrooms with Spinach and Feta
- Dessert: Peanut Butter and Banana Ice Cream

Day 30:

- Breakfast: Avocado and Spinach Omelette
- Lunch: Quinoa and Black Bean Stuffed Peppers
- Dinner: Baked Cod with Lemon and Herbs
- Snack: Guacamole with Veggie Sticks
- Dessert: Berry and Yogurt Popsicles

Chapter 2: Breakfast Recipes

In this chapter, we present a collection of breakfast recipes tailored for those navigating the path of diabetes. Bursting with wholesome ingredients and creative combinations, these recipes are designed to kickstart your day on a nutritious note.

Avocado and Spinach Omelette

Ingredients:

- 2 eggs
- 1/2 avocado, sliced
- Handful of fresh spinach
- Salt and pepper to taste

Instructions:

1. Whisk eggs in a bowl and season with salt and pepper.
2. Heat a non-stick pan and pour the egg mixture.
3. Add spinach and avocado slices.

4. Cook until the edges set, then flip and cook the other side.

5. Serve hot.

Nutrition Information (per serving):

- Calories: 250
- Protein: 15g
- Carbohydrates: 10g
- Fat: 18g
- Fiber: 6g
- Sugar: 1g
- Portion Size: 1 Omelette

Greek Yogurt Parfait with Berries

Ingredients:

- 1 cup Greek yogurt
- 1/2 cup mixed berries (strawberries, blueberries, raspberries)
- 1 tablespoon honey
- 1/4 cup granola

Instructions:

1. In a glass, layer Greek yogurt, berries, and granola.

2. Drizzle honey on top.

3. Repeat the layers.

4. Finish with a sprinkle of granola.

Nutrition Information (per serving):

- Calories: 300

- Protein: 20g

- Carbohydrates: 40g

- Fat: 8g

- Fiber: 5g

- Sugar: 18g

- Portion Size: 1 Parfait

Quinoa Breakfast Bowl

Ingredients:

- 1/2 cup cooked quinoa

- 1/4 cup almond milk

- 1/2 banana, sliced

- Handful of mixed nuts

- 1 teaspoon honey

Instructions:

1. Mix cooked quinoa with almond milk.
2. Top with banana slices, mixed nuts, and a drizzle of honey.
3. Stir and enjoy.

Nutrition Information (per serving):

- Calories: 280
- Protein: 10g
- Carbohydrates: 35g
- Fat: 12g
- Fiber: 5g
- Sugar: 10g
- Portion Size: 1 Bowl

Whole Grain Pancakes with Sugar-Free Syrup

Ingredients:

- 1 cup whole grain pancake mix
- 1 cup water
- Sugar-free syrup

Instructions:

1. Mix pancake mix with water.

2. Cook pancakes on a griddle.

3. Serve with sugar-free syrup.

Nutrition Information (per serving):

- Calories: 200

- Protein: 8g

- Carbohydrates: 40g

- Fat: 2g

- Fiber: 6g

- Sugar: 1g

- Portion Size: 2 Pancakes

Vegetable and Egg Breakfast Burrito

Ingredients:

- 1 whole-grain tortilla

- 2 eggs, scrambled

- 1/4 cup black beans

- Salsa and avocado for topping

Instructions:

1. Fill the tortilla with scrambled eggs and black beans.
2. Roll into a burrito.
3. Top with salsa and avocado.

Nutrition Information (per serving):

- Calories: 320
- Protein: 18g
- Carbohydrates: 30g
- Fat: 15g
- Fiber: 8g
- Sugar: 2g
- Portion Size: 1 Burrito

Chia Seed Pudding with Almonds

Ingredients:

- 2 tablespoons chia seeds
- 1/2 cup almond milk
- 1/4 teaspoon vanilla extract
- Sliced almonds for topping

Instructions:

1. Mix chia seeds, almond milk, and vanilla extract in a bowl.
2. Refrigerate overnight.
3. Top with sliced almonds before serving.

Nutrition Information (per serving):

- Calories: 180
- Protein: 5g
- Carbohydrates: 20g
- Fat: 10g
- Fiber: 8g
- Sugar: 2g
- Portion Size: 1 Pudding

Breakfast Casserole with Turkey Sausage

Ingredients:

- 6 eggs
- 1 cup turkey sausage, cooked and crumbled
- 1 cup spinach, chopped

- 1/2 cup low-fat cheese
- Salt and pepper to taste

Instructions:

1. Preheat the oven to 375°F (190°C).
2. In a bowl, whisk eggs and add cooked turkey sausage, spinach, and cheese.
3. Pour the mixture into a greased baking dish.
4. Bake for 25-30 minutes or until set.
5. Slice and serve.

Nutrition Information (per serving):

- Calories: 280
- Protein: 20g
- Carbohydrates: 5g
- Fat: 20g
- Fiber: 2g
- Sugar: 1g
- Portion Size: 1 Slice

Zucchini and Feta Muffins

Ingredients:

- 2 cups zucchini, grated
- 1/2 cup feta cheese, crumbled
- 1 cup whole wheat flour
- 1 teaspoon baking powder
- 2 eggs
- 1/4 cup olive oil

Instructions:

1. Preheat the oven to 350°F (175°C).
2. In a bowl, combine grated zucchini, feta, whole wheat flour, and baking powder.
3. In a separate bowl, whisk eggs and add olive oil.
4. Mix wet and dry ingredients.
5. Spoon into muffin cups and bake for 20-25 minutes.

Nutrition Information (per serving):

- Calories: 220
- Protein: 8g
- Carbohydrates: 15g
- Fat: 15g

- Fiber: 3g
- Sugar: 2g
- Portion Size: 1 Muffin

Smoked Salmon and Cream Cheese Bagel

Ingredients:

- 1 whole grain bagel
- 2 tablespoons cream cheese
- 2 ounces smoked salmon
- Fresh dill for garnish

Instructions:

1. Toast the whole grain bagel.
2. Spread cream cheese on the bagel halves.
3. Top with smoked salmon and fresh dill.

Nutrition Information (per serving):

- Calories: 320
- Protein: 20g
- Carbohydrates: 40g

- Fat: 10g

- Fiber: 5g

- Sugar: 2g

- Portion Size: 1 Bagel

Oatmeal with Walnuts and Berries

Ingredients:

- 1/2 cup rolled oats

- 1 cup water or milk

- 1/4 cup walnuts, chopped

- Handful of mixed berries

Instructions:

1. Cook rolled oats with water or milk.

2. Top with chopped walnuts and mixed berries.

Nutrition Information (per serving):

- Calories: 280

- Protein: 10g

- Carbohydrates: 35g

- Fat: 12g

- Fiber: 7g

- Sugar: 5g
- Portion Size: 1 Bowl

Cottage Cheese and Pineapple Bowl

Ingredients:

- 1 cup low-fat cottage cheese
- 1/2 cup fresh pineapple chunks
- 1 tablespoon shredded coconut

Instructions:

1. In a bowl, combine cottage cheese and fresh pineapple chunks.
2. Top with shredded coconut.

Nutrition Information (per serving):

- Calories: 220
- Protein: 20g
- Carbohydrates: 25g
- Fat: 5g
- Fiber: 2g
- Sugar: 18g
- Portion Size: 1 Bowl

Sweet Potato Hash with Poached Eggs

Ingredients:

- 1 sweet potato, diced
- 1 tablespoon olive oil
- 2 eggs, poached
- Salt and pepper to taste

Instructions:

1. Heat olive oil in a skillet and sauté diced sweet potato until cooked.
2. Season with salt and pepper.
3. Top with poached eggs.

Nutrition Information (per serving):

- Calories: 280
- Protein: 12g
- Carbohydrates: 30g
- Fat: 12g
- Fiber: 5g
- Sugar: 8g
- Portion Size: 1 Plate

Green Smoothie Bowl

Ingredients:

- 1 cup spinach
- 1/2 banana
- 1/2 cup pineapple chunks
- 1/2 cup almond milk
- Toppings: Chia seeds, sliced kiwi, and granola

Instructions:

1. Blend spinach, banana, pineapple, and almond milk until smooth.
2. Pour into a bowl and add toppings.

Nutrition Information (per serving):

- Calories: 200
- Protein: 5g
- Carbohydrates: 35g
- Fat: 7g
- Fiber: 8g
- Sugar: 18g
- Portion Size: 1 Bowl

Turkey and Vegetable Breakfast Wrap

Ingredients:

- 1 whole-grain tortilla
- 3 slices turkey breast
- 1/4 cup bell peppers, diced
- 2 eggs, scrambled

Instructions:

1. Warm the tortilla and layer with turkey slices.
2. Sauté diced bell peppers and scramble eggs.
3. Add the egg mixture to the tortilla, roll, and enjoy.

Nutrition Information (per serving):

- Calories: 300
- Protein: 20g
- Carbohydrates: 25g
- Fat: 15g
- Fiber: 5g
- Sugar: 2g
- Portion Size: 1 Wrap

Almond Butter and Banana Toast

Ingredients:

- 1 slice whole-grain bread
- 2 tablespoons almond butter
- 1/2 banana, sliced

Instructions:

1. Toast the whole-grain bread slice.
2. Spread almond butter on the toast.
3. Top with sliced bananas.

Nutrition Information (per serving):

- Calories: 250
- Protein: 8g
- Carbohydrates: 30g
- Fat: 12g
- Fiber: 6g
- Sugar: 10g
- Portion Size: 1 Slice

Chapter 3: Lunch Recipes

In this chapter, we delve into a collection of lunch recipes meticulously designed for individuals newly diagnosed with diabetes. These recipes not only prioritize health but also tantalize the taste buds with a symphony of flavors.

Grilled Chicken Salad with Balsamic Vinaigrette

Ingredients:

- 2 boneless, skinless chicken breasts
- 6 cups mixed salad greens
- 1 cup cherry tomatoes, halved
- 1 cucumber, sliced
- 1/4 cup red onion, thinly sliced
- 1/3 cup balsamic vinaigrette dressing

Instructions:

1. Preheat the grill to medium-high heat.
2. Season chicken breasts with salt and pepper.

3. Grill chicken for 6-8 minutes per side until fully cooked.

4. Let chicken rest, then slice into strips.

5. In a large bowl, combine salad greens, cherry tomatoes, cucumber, and red onion.

6. Top with grilled chicken strips.

7. Drizzle with balsamic vinaigrette and toss gently.

8. Serve immediately.

Nutrition Information (per serving):

- Calories: 320
- Protein: 28g
- Carbohydrates: 15g
- Fat: 15g
- Fiber: 5g
- Sugar: 8g
- Portion Size: 1 serving

Quinoa and Black Bean Stuffed Peppers

Ingredients:

- 4 large bell peppers, halved and seeds removed
- 1 cup cooked quinoa
- 1 can (15 oz) black beans, drained and rinsed
- 1 cup corn kernels
- 1 cup diced tomatoes
- 1 teaspoon cumin
- 1 teaspoon chili powder
- 1/2 cup shredded cheddar cheese (optional)

Instructions:

1. Preheat the oven to 375°F (190°C).
2. In a large bowl, mix cooked quinoa, black beans, corn, diced tomatoes, cumin, and chili powder.
3. Spoon the mixture into halved bell peppers.
4. If desired, sprinkle shredded cheddar cheese on top.
5. Place stuffed peppers in a baking dish.
6. Bake for 25-30 minutes or until peppers are tender.
7. Serve warm.

Nutrition Information (per serving):

- Calories: 280
- Protein: 12g
- Carbohydrates: 48g
- Fat: 5g
- Fiber: 10g
- Sugar: 6g
- Portion Size: 1/2 stuffed pepper

Salmon and Asparagus Foil Pack

Ingredients:

- 2 salmon fillets
- 1 bunch asparagus, trimmed
- 1 lemon, sliced
- 2 tablespoons olive oil
- 1 teaspoon garlic powder
- Salt and pepper to taste

Instructions:

1. Preheat the oven to 400°F (200°C).
2. Place each salmon fillet on a piece of foil.
3. Arrange asparagus around the salmon.

4. Drizzle olive oil over salmon and asparagus.

5. Sprinkle garlic powder, salt, and pepper.

6. Place lemon slices on top.

7. Fold the foil to create a packet.

8. Bake for 20-25 minutes or until salmon flakes easily.

9. Serve with a wedge of lemon.

Nutrition Information (per serving):

- Calories: 350
- Protein: 25g
- Carbohydrates: 10g
- Fat: 23g
- Fiber: 4g
- Sugar: 2g
- Portion Size: 1 serving

Turkey and Vegetable Stir-Fry

Ingredients:

- 1 lb lean ground turkey
- 2 cups broccoli florets
- 1 bell pepper, sliced
- 1 cup snap peas

- 2 carrots, julienned
- 3 tablespoons low-sodium soy sauce
- 1 tablespoon sesame oil
- 1 teaspoon ginger, minced
- 2 cloves garlic, minced

Instructions:

1. In a large skillet, brown ground turkey over medium heat.
2. Add broccoli, bell pepper, snap peas, and carrots.
3. In a small bowl, whisk together soy sauce, sesame oil, ginger, and garlic.
4. Pour sauce over the turkey and vegetables.
5. Stir-fry until vegetables are tender-crisp.
6. Serve over brown rice or quinoa.

Nutrition Information (per serving):

- Calories: 320
- Protein: 28g
- Carbohydrates: 20g
- Fat: 15g
- Fiber: 6g

- Sugar: 8g
- Portion Size: 1 cup stir-fry

Lentil Soup with Vegetables

Ingredients:

- 1 cup dried green lentils, rinsed
- 1 onion, chopped
- 2 carrots, diced
- 2 celery stalks, sliced
- 3 cloves garlic, minced
- 6 cups vegetable broth
- 1 can (14 oz) diced tomatoes
- 1 teaspoon cumin
- 1 teaspoon thyme
- Salt and pepper to taste

Instructions:

1. In a large pot, sauté onion, carrots, and celery until softened.
2. Add garlic and cook for an additional minute.
3. Stir in lentils, vegetable broth, diced tomatoes, cumin, thyme, salt, and pepper.

4. Bring to a boil, then reduce heat and simmer for 25-30 minutes.

5. Adjust seasoning if necessary.

6. Serve hot.

Nutrition Information (per serving):

- Calories: 220

- Protein: 14g

- Carbohydrates: 38g

- Fat: 1g

- Fiber: 15g

- Sugar: 5g

- Portion Size: 1 cup

Caprese Salad with Chicken

Ingredients:

- 2 boneless, skinless chicken breasts

- 2 cups cherry tomatoes, halved

- 1 cup fresh mozzarella, diced

- 1/4 cup fresh basil, chopped

- 2 tablespoons balsamic glaze

- Salt and pepper to taste

Instructions:

1. Season chicken breasts with salt and pepper.
2. Grill or pan-cook chicken until fully cooked.
3. Slice chicken into thin strips.
4. In a bowl, combine cherry tomatoes, fresh mozzarella, and fresh basil.
5. Add sliced chicken on top.
6. Drizzle with balsamic glaze.
7. Toss gently and serve.

Nutrition Information (per serving):

- Calories: 320
- Protein: 32g
- Carbohydrates: 10g
- Fat: 15g
- Fiber: 2g
- Sugar: 5g
- Portion Size: 1 serving

Whole Grain Wrap with Hummus and Vegetables

Ingredients:

- 4 whole grain wraps
- 1 cup hummus
- 2 cups mixed salad greens
- 1 cucumber, julienned
- 1 bell pepper, sliced
- 1/2 red onion, thinly sliced

Instructions:

1. Spread a generous layer of hummus on each whole grain wrap.
2. Layer with mixed salad greens, cucumber, bell pepper, and red onion.
3. Roll the wraps tightly, folding in the sides.
4. Slice in half and secure with toothpicks if needed.
5. Serve immediately.

Nutrition Information (per serving):

- Calories: 280
- Protein: 10g

- Carbohydrates: 40g

- Fat: 10g

- Fiber: 8g

- Sugar: 5g

- Portion Size: 1 wrap

Shrimp and Quinoa Bowl

Ingredients:

- 1 lb shrimp, peeled and deveined

- 2 cups cooked quinoa

- 1 cup cherry tomatoes, halved

- 1 avocado, diced

- 1/4 cup cilantro, chopped

- 1 lime, juiced

- Salt and pepper to taste

Instructions:

1. Season shrimp with salt and pepper.

2. In a skillet, cook shrimp until pink and opaque.

3. In a bowl, combine cooked quinoa, cherry tomatoes, avocado, and cilantro.

4. Top with cooked shrimp.

5. Drizzle with lime juice.

6. Toss gently and serve.

Nutrition Information (per serving):

- Calories: 340

- Protein: 30g

- Carbohydrates: 30g

- Fat: 15g

- Fiber: 7g

- Sugar: 3g

- Portion Size: 1 cup

Chickpea and Spinach Salad

Ingredients:

- 2 cups canned chickpeas, drained and rinsed

- 3 cups fresh spinach

- 1 cup cherry tomatoes, halved

- 1/2 red onion, thinly sliced

- 1/4 cup feta cheese, crumbled

- 2 tablespoons olive oil

- 1 tablespoon balsamic vinegar

- Salt and pepper to taste

Instructions:

1. In a large bowl, combine chickpeas, spinach, cherry tomatoes, red onion, and feta cheese.
2. Drizzle with olive oil and balsamic vinegar.
3. Season with salt and pepper.
4. Toss gently and serve.

Nutrition Information (per serving):

- Calories: 280
- Protein: 14g
- Carbohydrates: 35g
- Fat: 10g
- Fiber: 8g
- Sugar: 6g
- Portion Size: 1 cup

Turkey and Avocado Wrap

Ingredients:

- 1 lb sliced turkey breast
- 4 whole wheat wraps
- 1 avocado, sliced
- 1 cup shredded lettuce

- 1/2 cup cherry tomatoes, halved
- 2 tablespoons Greek yogurt
- Salt and pepper to taste

Instructions:

1. Lay out the whole wheat wraps.
2. Layer with turkey slices, avocado, shredded lettuce, and cherry tomatoes.
3. Drizzle Greek yogurt over the ingredients.
4. Sprinkle with salt and pepper.
5. Roll the wraps tightly, folding in the sides.
6. Slice in half and secure with toothpicks if needed.
7. Serve immediately.

Nutrition Information (per serving):

- Calories: 320
- Protein: 25g
- Carbohydrates: 30g
- Fat: 12g
- Fiber: 7g
- Sugar: 3g
- Portion Size: 1 wrap

Vegetable and Tofu Stir-Fry

Ingredients:

- 1 block firm tofu, cubed
- 2 tablespoons soy sauce
- 1 tablespoon sesame oil
- 1 tablespoon cornstarch
- 2 tablespoons vegetable oil
- 2 cups broccoli florets
- 1 bell pepper, sliced
- 1 cup snow peas
- 1 carrot, julienned
- 2 cloves garlic, minced
- 1 tablespoon ginger, minced

Instructions:

1. In a bowl, toss tofu cubes with soy sauce, sesame oil, and cornstarch.
2. Heat vegetable oil in a wok or skillet.
3. Add tofu and cook until golden brown.
4. Remove tofu from the pan.

5. In the same pan, stir-fry broccoli, bell pepper, snow peas, carrot, garlic, and ginger until vegetables are tender-crisp.

6. Add cooked tofu back to the pan and toss.

7. Serve over brown rice or quinoa.

Nutrition Information (per serving):

- Calories: 290
- Protein: 18g
- Carbohydrates: 20g
- Fat: 15g
- Fiber: 6g
- Sugar: 4g
- Portion Size: 1 cup stir-fry

Mediterranean Quinoa Salad

Ingredients:

- 2 cups cooked quinoa
- 1 cup cucumber, diced
- 1 cup cherry tomatoes, halved
- 1/2 cup Kalamata olives, sliced
- 1/4 cup red onion, finely chopped

- 1/2 cup feta cheese, crumbled
- 2 tablespoons olive oil
- 1 tablespoon red wine vinegar
- 1 teaspoon dried oregano
- Salt and pepper to taste

Instructions:

1. In a large bowl, combine cooked quinoa, cucumber, cherry tomatoes, Kalamata olives, red onion, and feta cheese.
2. In a small bowl, whisk together olive oil, red wine vinegar, dried oregano, salt, and pepper.
3. Pour the dressing over the salad and toss gently.
4. Serve chilled.

Nutrition Information (per serving):

- Calories: 320
- Protein: 12g
- Carbohydrates: 30g
- Fat: 18g
- Fiber: 5g
- Sugar: 3g

- Portion Size: 1 cup

Spinach and Feta Turkey Burger

Ingredients:

- 1 lb ground turkey
- 2 cups fresh spinach, chopped
- 1/2 cup feta cheese, crumbled
- 1/4 cup red onion, finely chopped
- 1 teaspoon garlic powder
- Salt and pepper to taste
- Whole wheat burger buns

Instructions:

1. In a large bowl, combine ground turkey, chopped spinach, feta cheese, red onion, garlic powder, salt, and pepper.
2. Mix until ingredients are well incorporated.
3. Form the mixture into burger patties.
4. Grill or pan-cook the turkey burgers until fully cooked.
5. Toast whole wheat burger buns.
6. Place turkey burgers on the buns.

7. Serve with your favorite toppings.

Nutrition Information (per serving):

- Calories: 280
- Protein: 24g
- Carbohydrates: 20g
- Fat: 12g
- Fiber: 3g
- Sugar: 2g
- Portion Size: 1 burger

Chicken Caesar Salad with Whole Grain Croutons

Ingredients:

- 2 boneless, skinless chicken breasts
- 6 cups romaine lettuce, chopped
- 1/2 cup cherry tomatoes, halved
- 1/4 cup Parmesan cheese, grated
- Whole grain croutons
- Caesar dressing (low-fat)

Instructions:

1. Season chicken breasts with salt and pepper.
2. Grill or pan-cook chicken until fully cooked.
3. Let chicken rest, then slice into thin strips.
4. In a large bowl, combine chopped romaine lettuce, cherry tomatoes, Parmesan cheese, and chicken strips.
5. Toss with whole grain croutons.
6. Drizzle with Caesar dressing and toss gently.
7. Serve immediately.

Nutrition Information (per serving):

- Calories: 320
- Protein: 28g
- Carbohydrates: 15g
- Fat: 15g
- Fiber: 5g
- Sugar: 3g
- Portion Size: 1 serving

Eggplant and Tomato Stack

Ingredients:

- 2 large eggplants, sliced
- 4 large tomatoes, sliced
- 1 cup mozzarella cheese, shredded
- 1/4 cup fresh basil leaves
- 2 tablespoons olive oil
- Balsamic glaze for drizzling
- Salt and pepper to taste

Instructions:

1. Preheat the oven to 375°F (190°C).
2. Place eggplant slices on a baking sheet.
3. Drizzle with olive oil, salt, and pepper.
4. Bake for 20-25 minutes or until eggplant is tender.
5. In a separate baking dish, layer sliced tomatoes, mozzarella cheese, and fresh basil leaves.
6. Top with roasted eggplant slices.
7. Bake for an additional 15 minutes or until cheese is melted and bubbly.
8. Drizzle with balsamic glaze before serving.

Nutrition Information (per serving):

- Calories: 250
- Protein: 10g
- Carbohydrates: 20g
- Fat: 15g
- Fiber: 8g
- Sugar: 10g
- Portion Size: 1 stack

Chapter 4: Dinner Recipes

In this chapter, you'll find delicious and diabetes-friendly dinner recipes that prioritize taste, nutrition, and ease of preparation. Each recipe includes clear instructions, a list of ingredients, and nutritional information to assist you in making informed choices.

Baked Cod with Lemon and Herbs

Ingredients:

- 4 cod fillets
- 1 lemon (juiced and zested)
- 2 tablespoons olive oil
- 2 cloves garlic (minced)
- 1 teaspoon dried oregano
- Salt and pepper to taste

Instructions:

1. Preheat the oven to 375°F (190°C).
2. In a small bowl, mix lemon juice, lemon zest, olive oil, minced garlic, dried oregano, salt, and pepper.

3. Place the cod fillets in a baking dish and pour the lemon and herb mixture over them.

4. Bake for 15-20 minutes or until the cod is opaque and flakes easily with a fork.

5. Serve hot.

Nutrition Information (per serving):

- Calories: 200

- Protein: 25g

- Carbohydrates: 2g

- Fat: 10g

- Fiber: 0.5g

- Sugar: 0.5g

- Portion Size: 1 fillet

Cauliflower Rice and Chicken Curry

Ingredients:

- 2 cups cauliflower rice

- 1 lb boneless, skinless chicken breasts (cubed)

- 1 can coconut milk

- 2 tablespoons curry powder

- 1 onion (diced)

- 2 cloves garlic (minced)
- Salt and pepper to taste

Instructions:

1. In a pan, sauté diced onion and minced garlic until softened.
2. Add chicken cubes and cook until browned.
3. Stir in curry powder and pour in coconut milk.
4. Simmer for 15-20 minutes until the chicken is cooked through.
5. Serve the curry over cauliflower rice.

Nutrition Information (per serving):

- Calories: 300
- Protein: 30g
- Carbohydrates: 10g
- Fat: 15g
- Fiber: 3g
- Sugar: 3g
- Portion Size: 1 cup

Beef and Vegetable Skewers

Ingredients:

- 1 lb lean beef cubes
- 1 bell pepper (cut into chunks)
- 1 zucchini (sliced)
- 1 red onion (cut into wedges)
- 2 tablespoons olive oil
- 1 teaspoon smoked paprika
- Salt and pepper to taste

Instructions:

1. Preheat the grill or oven to medium-high heat.
2. In a bowl, toss beef cubes, bell pepper, zucchini, red onion, olive oil, smoked paprika, salt, and pepper.
3. Thread the marinated ingredients onto skewers.
4. Grill for 10-15 minutes, turning occasionally, until the beef is cooked to your liking.
5. Serve hot.

Nutrition Information (per serving):

- Calories: 250
- Protein: 25g

- Carbohydrates: 5g

- Fat: 15g

- Fiber: 2g

- Sugar: 3g

- Portion Size: 2 skewers

Stuffed Bell Peppers with Ground Turkey

Ingredients:

- 4 bell peppers (halved and seeds removed)

- 1 lb ground turkey

- 1 cup cooked quinoa

- 1 can diced tomatoes

- 1 teaspoon cumin

- 1 teaspoon chili powder

- Salt and pepper to taste

Instructions:

1. Preheat the oven to 375°F (190°C).

2. In a skillet, brown the ground turkey. Drain excess fat.

3. Mix in cooked quinoa, diced tomatoes, cumin, chili powder, salt, and pepper.
4. Stuff each bell pepper half with the turkey mixture.
5. Bake for 25-30 minutes until peppers are tender.

Nutrition Information (per serving):

- Calories: 280
- Protein: 20g
- Carbohydrates: 20g
- Fat: 10g
- Fiber: 4g
- Sugar: 6g
- Portion Size: 2 pepper halves

Grilled Veggie and Quinoa Stuffed Portobello Mushrooms

Ingredients:

- 4 large Portobello mushrooms
- 1 cup cooked quinoa
- 1 zucchini (diced)
- 1 red bell pepper (diced)

- 2 tablespoons balsamic vinegar
- 2 tablespoons olive oil
- 1 teaspoon dried thyme
- Salt and pepper to taste

Instructions:

1. Preheat the grill or oven to medium-high heat.
2. Remove the stems from Portobello mushrooms and brush with olive oil.
3. In a bowl, mix cooked quinoa, diced zucchini, diced red bell pepper, balsamic vinegar, olive oil, dried thyme, salt, and pepper.
4. Stuff each mushroom with the quinoa mixture.
5. Grill for 15-20 minutes until mushrooms are tender.

Nutrition Information (per serving):

- Calories: 220
- Protein: 8g
- Carbohydrates: 30g
- Fat: 8g
- Fiber: 5g
- Sugar: 5g

- Portion Size: 1 stuffed mushroom

Zoodle (Zucchini Noodle) Lasagna

Ingredients:

- 4 medium zucchinis (spiralized into noodles)
- 1 lb lean ground beef
- 1 can crushed tomatoes
- 1 cup part-skim ricotta cheese
- 1 cup shredded mozzarella cheese
- 1 teaspoon Italian seasoning
- Salt and pepper to taste

Instructions:

1. Preheat the oven to 375°F (190°C).
2. In a skillet, brown the ground beef. Drain excess fat.
3. Add crushed tomatoes, Italian seasoning, salt, and pepper. Simmer for 10 minutes.
4. In a baking dish, layer zucchini noodles, meat sauce, ricotta, and mozzarella. Repeat.
5. Bake for 30-35 minutes until the top is golden and bubbly.

Nutrition Information (per serving):

- Calories: 320
- Protein: 25g
- Carbohydrates: 15g
- Fat: 18g
- Fiber: 5g
- Sugar: 8g
- Portion Size: 1 slice

Lemon Garlic Roast Chicken

Ingredients:

- 4 chicken thighs (bone-in, skin-on)
- 2 lemons (juiced and zested)
- 4 cloves garlic (minced)
- 2 tablespoons olive oil
- 1 teaspoon dried rosemary
- Salt and pepper to taste

Instructions:

1. Preheat the oven to 400°F (200°C).
2. In a bowl, mix lemon juice, lemon zest, minced garlic, olive oil, dried rosemary, salt, and pepper.

3. Rub the chicken thighs with the lemon and garlic mixture.

4. Roast in the oven for 40-45 minutes until the chicken is golden and juices run clear.

5. Serve hot.

Nutrition Information (per serving):

- Calories: 280
- Protein: 30g
- Carbohydrates: 4g
- Fat: 16g
- Fiber: 1g
- Sugar: 1g
- Portion Size: 1 chicken thigh

Spaghetti Squash with Turkey Meatballs

Ingredients:

- 1 medium spaghetti squash (halved and seeds removed)
- 1 lb lean ground turkey

- 1 can crushed tomatoes
- 1 teaspoon Italian seasoning
- 1 egg
- 1/4 cup grated Parmesan cheese
- Salt and pepper to taste

Instructions:

1. Preheat the oven to 375°F (190°C).
2. Place spaghetti squash halves on a baking sheet, cut side down. Roast for 40-45 minutes until tender.
3. In a bowl, mix ground turkey, crushed tomatoes, Italian seasoning, egg, Parmesan cheese, salt, and pepper. Form into meatballs.
4. Bake meatballs at 375°F (190°C) for 20-25 minutes.
5. Scrape the cooked spaghetti squash with a fork to create "noodles" and serve with turkey meatballs.

Nutrition Information (per serving):

- Calories: 280
- Protein: 25g
- Carbohydrates: 20g
- Fat: 12g

- Fiber: 5g

- Sugar: 8g

- Portion Size: 1 cup spaghetti squash with 3 meatballs

Teriyaki Salmon with Broccoli

Ingredients:

- 4 salmon fillets

- 1/2 cup low-sodium teriyaki sauce

- 2 tablespoons honey

- 1 tablespoon sesame oil

- 2 cups broccoli florets

- Sesame seeds for garnish

Instructions:

1. Preheat the oven to 400°F (200°C).

2. In a bowl, mix teriyaki sauce, honey, and sesame oil.

3. Place salmon fillets on a baking sheet and brush with the teriyaki mixture.

4. Toss broccoli in the remaining teriyaki mixture and arrange around the salmon.

5. Bake for 15-20 minutes until salmon is cooked through and broccoli is tender.

6. Garnish with sesame seeds and serve.

Nutrition Information (per serving):

- Calories: 320
- Protein: 25g
- Carbohydrates: 18g
- Fat: 15g
- Fiber: 3g
- Sugar: 12g
- Portion Size: 1 salmon fillet with broccoli

Sweet Potato and Black Bean Chili

Ingredients:

- 2 sweet potatoes (peeled and diced)
- 1 can black beans (drained and rinsed)
- 1 lb lean ground turkey
- 1 can diced tomatoes
- 2 tablespoons chili powder
- 1 teaspoon cumin
- Salt and pepper to taste

Instructions:

1. In a large pot, brown the ground turkey.
2. Add diced sweet potatoes, black beans, diced tomatoes, chili powder, cumin, salt, and pepper.
3. Simmer for 20-25 minutes until sweet potatoes are tender.
4. Serve hot.

Nutrition Information (per serving):

- Calories: 300
- Protein: 25g
- Carbohydrates: 35g
- Fat: 8g
- Fiber: 10g
- Sugar: 8g
- Portion Size: 1 cup

Ratatouille with Chickpeas

Ingredients:

- 1 eggplant (sliced)
- 2 zucchinis (sliced)
- 1 bell pepper (sliced)

- 1 onion (sliced)
- 2 tomatoes (sliced)
- 1 can chickpeas (drained and rinsed)
- 2 tablespoons olive oil
- 2 cloves garlic (minced)
- 1 teaspoon dried thyme
- Salt and pepper to taste

Instructions:

1. Preheat the oven to 375°F (190°C).
2. In a baking dish, layer sliced eggplant, zucchini, bell pepper, onion, and tomatoes.
3. Sprinkle chickpeas over the vegetables.
4. In a bowl, mix olive oil, minced garlic, dried thyme, salt, and pepper. Drizzle over the vegetables.
5. Bake for 40-45 minutes until the vegetables are tender.

Nutrition Information (per serving):

- Calories: 250
- Protein: 8g
- Carbohydrates: 35g

- Fat: 10g
- Fiber: 10g
- Sugar: 10g
- Portion Size: 1 cup

Pesto Zucchini Noodles with Cherry Tomatoes

Ingredients:

- 4 medium zucchinis (spiralized into noodles)
- 1 cup cherry tomatoes (halved)
- 1/2 cup basil pesto
- 1/4 cup grated Parmesan cheese
- 2 tablespoons pine nuts (toasted)
- Salt and pepper to taste

Instructions:

1. In a skillet, sauté zucchini noodles until slightly softened.
2. Toss in cherry tomatoes and cook for an additional 2-3 minutes.

3. Stir in basil pesto, Parmesan cheese, and toasted pine nuts.

4. Cook for an additional 2 minutes until heated through.

5. Serve warm.

Nutrition Information (per serving):

- Calories: 280
- Protein: 8g
- Carbohydrates: 15g
- Fat: 22g
- Fiber: 4g
- Sugar: 8g
- Portion Size: 1 cup

Turkey and Vegetable Lettuce Wraps

Ingredients:

- 1 lb ground turkey
- 1 cup shredded carrots
- 1 cup diced bell peppers

- 1/2 cup hoisin sauce
- 2 tablespoons soy sauce
- 1 teaspoon sesame oil
- 1 head iceberg lettuce (leaves separated)

Instructions:

1. In a skillet, brown the ground turkey.
2. Add shredded carrots and diced bell peppers. Cook until vegetables are tender.
3. Stir in hoisin sauce, soy sauce, and sesame oil.
4. Spoon the turkey and vegetable mixture into lettuce leaves.
5. Serve as wraps.

Nutrition Information (per serving):

- Calories: 240
- Protein: 20g
- Carbohydrates: 15g
- Fat: 12g
- Fiber: 4g
- Sugar: 8g
- Portion Size: 2 wraps

BBQ Chicken and Vegetable Skewers

Ingredients:

- 1 lb boneless, skinless chicken breasts (cut into chunks)
- 2 bell peppers (cut into chunks)
- 1 red onion (cut into wedges)
- 1 zucchini (sliced)
- 1/2 cup BBQ sauce
- 2 tablespoons olive oil
- 1 teaspoon smoked paprika
- Salt and pepper to taste

Instructions:

1. Preheat the grill or oven to medium-high heat.
2. In a bowl, mix chicken chunks, bell peppers, red onion, zucchini, BBQ sauce, olive oil, smoked paprika, salt, and pepper.
3. Thread the marinated ingredients onto skewers.
4. Grill for 12-15 minutes, turning occasionally, until chicken is cooked through.
5. Serve hot.

Nutrition Information (per serving):

- Calories: 280
- Protein: 25g
- Carbohydrates: 20g
- Fat: 10g
- Fiber: 4g
- Sugar: 10g
- Portion Size: 2 skewers

Creamy Mushroom and Spinach Risotto

Ingredients:

- 1 cup Arborio rice
- 4 cups vegetable broth (low sodium)
- 1 cup mushrooms (sliced)
- 2 cups fresh spinach
- 1/2 cup Parmesan cheese (grated)
- 2 tablespoons olive oil
- 1 onion (finely chopped)
- 2 cloves garlic (minced)
- Salt and pepper to taste

Instructions:

1. In a saucepan, heat olive oil over medium heat. Add chopped onion and minced garlic. Sauté until softened.
2. Add Arborio rice and cook for 2-3 minutes until lightly toasted.
3. Gradually add vegetable broth, one ladle at a time, stirring constantly until absorbed.
4. Stir in sliced mushrooms and continue adding broth until rice is creamy and cooked to al dente.
5. Fold in fresh spinach and Parmesan cheese. Season with salt and pepper.
6. Serve hot.

Nutrition Information (per serving):

- Calories: 300
- Protein: 10g
- Carbohydrates: 40g
- Fat: 12g
- Fiber: 3g
- Sugar: 2g
- Portion Size: 1 cup

Chapter 5: Snacks and Appetizers

In this chapter, we present a collection of Snacks and Appetizers crafted with wholesome ingredients and thoughtful combinations. Embrace these delicious options without compromising on your health goals.

Guacamole with Veggie Sticks

Ingredients:

- 2 ripe avocados
- 1 medium tomato, diced
- 1/4 cup red onion, finely chopped
- 1 clove garlic, minced
- 1 lime, juiced
- Salt and pepper to taste
- Veggie sticks (carrots, bell peppers, cucumber) for dipping

Instructions:

1. In a bowl, mash avocados with a fork.

2. Add diced tomato, red onion, minced garlic, and lime juice. Mix well.

3. Season with salt and pepper to taste.

4. Serve with veggie sticks for a crunchy and satisfying snack.

Nutrition Information (per serving):

- Calories: 120

- Protein: 2g

- Carbohydrates: 8g

- Fat: 10g

- Fiber: 5g

- Sugar: 1g

- Portion size: 1/2 cup guacamole with veggie sticks

Greek Yogurt and Berry Parfait

Ingredients:

- 1 cup Greek yogurt

- 1/2 cup mixed berries (strawberries, blueberries, raspberries)

- 2 tablespoons honey

- Granola for layering

Instructions:

1. In a glass, layer Greek yogurt, mixed berries, and a drizzle of honey.
2. Repeat the layers until the glass is filled.
3. Top with granola for added crunch and texture.
4. Enjoy this delightful parfait as a nutritious snack.

Nutrition Information (per serving):

- Calories: 180
- Protein: 15g
- Carbohydrates: 25g
- Fat: 3g
- Fiber: 4g
- Sugar: 18g
- Portion size: 1 parfait

Hummus and Whole Grain Crackers

Ingredients:

- 1 cup hummus
- Whole grain crackers for dipping

Instructions:

1. Place hummus in a serving bowl.

2. Arrange whole grain crackers around the bowl.

3. Dip and enjoy the creamy texture of hummus with the wholesome crunch of whole grain crackers.

Nutrition Information (per serving):

- Calories: 150

- Protein: 5g

- Carbohydrates: 20g

- Fat: 7g

- Fiber: 5g

- Sugar: 1g

- Portion size: 1/2 cup hummus with crackers

Cheese and Grape Skewers

Ingredients:

- Cubes of your favorite cheese (cheddar, mozzarella, or goat cheese)

- Fresh grapes

Instructions:

1. Skewer a cube of cheese followed by a grape onto toothpicks or small skewers.
2. Repeat until you have a delightful arrangement.
3. Serve these sweet and savory skewers for a sophisticated snack.

Nutrition Information (per serving):

- Calories: 120
- Protein: 8g
- Carbohydrates: 10g
- Fat: 6g
- Fiber: 1g
- Sugar: 6g
- Portion size: 5 skewers

Roasted Chickpeas with Paprika

Ingredients:

- 1 can (15 oz) chickpeas, drained and rinsed
- 1 tablespoon olive oil
- 1 teaspoon paprika
- Salt to taste

Instructions:

1. Preheat the oven to 400°F (200°C).

2. Pat the chickpeas dry and toss them in a bowl with olive oil, paprika, and salt.

3. Spread the chickpeas on a baking sheet and roast for 20-25 minutes until crispy.

4. Allow them to cool before indulging in this protein-packed and flavorful snack.

Nutrition Information (per serving):

- Calories: 150
- Protein: 6g
- Carbohydrates: 22g
- Fat: 5g
- Fiber: 6g
- Sugar: 4g
- Portion size: 1/2 cup roasted chickpeas

Cucumber and Tomato Salsa

Ingredients:

- 1 cucumber, diced
- 1 cup cherry tomatoes, halved

- 1/4 cup red onion, finely chopped
- 1/4 cup fresh cilantro, chopped
- 1 jalapeño, seeded and minced (optional)
- 1 lime, juiced
- Salt and pepper to taste

Instructions:

1. In a bowl, combine cucumber, cherry tomatoes, red onion, cilantro, and jalapeño.
2. Squeeze lime juice over the mixture and season with salt and pepper.
3. Stir well and refrigerate for at least 30 minutes before serving.
4. Enjoy this refreshing salsa with whole wheat pita chips or as a topping for grilled chicken.

Nutrition Information (per serving):

- Calories: 40
- Protein: 1g
- Carbohydrates: 10g
- Fat: 0g
- Fiber: 2g

- Sugar: 4g
- Portion size: 1/2 cup salsa

Apple Slices with Almond Butter

Ingredients:

- 2 apples, thinly sliced
- 1/4 cup almond butter

Instructions:

1. Arrange apple slices on a plate.
2. Microwave almond butter for 15-20 seconds to soften.
3. Drizzle almond butter over the apple slices.
4. Savor the combination of crisp apples and creamy almond butter for a wholesome treat.

Nutrition Information (per serving):

- Calories: 180
- Protein: 4g
- Carbohydrates: 25g
- Fat: 8g
- Fiber: 6g

- Sugar: 18g
- Portion size: 1 apple with almond butter

Edamame with Sea Salt

Ingredients:

- 1 cup edamame (frozen or fresh)
- Sea salt to taste

Instructions:

1. Boil or steam edamame according to package instructions.
2. Sprinkle with sea salt and toss to coat.
3. Enjoy these protein-rich and lightly salted edamame pods as a satisfying and nutritious snack.

Nutrition Information (per serving):

- Calories: 120
- Protein: 11g
- Carbohydrates: 9g
- Fat: 5g
- Fiber: 6g
- Sugar: 2g

- Portion size: 1 cup edamame

Caprese Kabobs with Balsamic Glaze

Ingredients:

- Cherry tomatoes
- Fresh mozzarella balls
- Basil leaves
- Balsamic glaze for drizzling

Instructions:

1. Thread a cherry tomato, a mozzarella ball, and a basil leaf onto toothpicks or small skewers.
2. Arrange the Caprese kabobs on a serving platter.
3. Drizzle with balsamic glaze just before serving.
4. Delight in the classic flavors of Caprese in a convenient and bite-sized form.

Nutrition Information (per serving):

- Calories: 90
- Protein: 5g

- Carbohydrates: 4g
- Fat: 6g
- Fiber: 1g
- Sugar: 2g
- Portion size: 5 kabobs

Trail Mix with Nuts and Dried Fruit

Ingredients:

- 1/2 cup almonds
- 1/2 cup walnuts
- 1/4 cup dried cranberries
- 1/4 cup raisins
- 1/4 cup dark chocolate chips

Instructions:

1. Mix almonds, walnuts, dried cranberries, raisins, and dark chocolate chips in a bowl.
2. Portion the trail mix into snack-sized bags for a convenient grab-and-go option.
3. Enjoy this energy-boosting mix of nuts and dried fruit whenever hunger strikes.

Nutrition Information (per serving):

- Calories: 200
- Protein: 6g
- Carbohydrates: 18g
- Fat: 14g
- Fiber: 4g
- Sugar: 9g
- Portion size: 1/2 cup trail mix

Veggie Spring Rolls with Peanut Sauce

Ingredients:

- Rice paper wrappers
- Shredded cabbage
- Carrots, julienned
- Cucumber, julienned
- Bell peppers, thinly sliced
- Fresh mint leaves
- Peanut sauce for dipping

Instructions:

1. Soften rice paper wrappers in warm water.

2. Place a small amount of shredded cabbage, carrots, cucumber, bell peppers, and mint on each wrapper.

3. Fold in the sides and roll tightly.

4. Serve with peanut sauce for a light and refreshing snack.

Nutrition Information (per serving):

- Calories: 120

- Protein: 3g

- Carbohydrates: 25g

- Fat: 1g

- Fiber: 4g

- Sugar: 4g

- Portion size: 2 spring rolls with peanut sauce

Cottage Cheese and Pineapple Skewers

Ingredients:

- Cottage cheese

- Fresh pineapple chunks

Instructions:

1. Thread cottage cheese and pineapple chunks onto toothpicks or small skewers.
2. Chill in the refrigerator before serving for a refreshing and protein-packed snack.
3. Enjoy the sweet and savory combination of cottage cheese and pineapple.

Nutrition Information (per serving):

- Calories: 90
- Protein: 10g
- Carbohydrates: 10g
- Fat: 1g
- Fiber: 1g
- Sugar: 7g
- Portion size: 5 skewers

Stuffed Mushrooms with Spinach and Feta

Ingredients:

- Button mushrooms, stems removed
- Spinach, chopped
- Feta cheese, crumbled
- Garlic, minced
- Olive oil
- Salt and pepper to taste

Instructions:

1. Preheat the oven to 375°F (190°C).
2. In a skillet, sauté spinach and garlic in olive oil until wilted.
3. Fill each mushroom cap with the spinach mixture and top with crumbled feta.
4. Bake for 15-20 minutes until mushrooms are tender.
5. Enjoy these savory stuffed mushrooms as a flavorful appetizer.

Nutrition Information (per serving):

- Calories: 80

- Protein: 4g

- Carbohydrates: 5g

- Fat: 6g

- Fiber: 2g

- Sugar: 2g

- Portion size: 5 stuffed mushrooms

Avocado and Tomato Bruschetta

Ingredients:

- Baguette slices, toasted

- Ripe avocados, mashed

- Cherry tomatoes, diced

- Red onion, finely chopped

- Fresh basil, chopped

- Balsamic glaze for drizzling

Instructions:

1. Spread mashed avocado on toasted baguette slices.

2. Top with diced tomatoes, red onion, and fresh basil.

3. Drizzle with balsamic glaze before serving.

4. Enjoy this delightful bruschetta with a burst of flavors.

Nutrition Information (per serving):

- Calories: 110
- Protein: 2g
- Carbohydrates: 15g
- Fat: 5g
- Fiber: 4g
- Sugar: 2g
- Portion size: 4 bruschetta slices

Spinach and Artichoke Dip with Whole Wheat Pita

Ingredients:

- 1 cup frozen chopped spinach, thawed and drained
- 1 can (14 oz) artichoke hearts, drained and chopped
- 1 cup Greek yogurt
- 1/2 cup mayonnaise
- 1 cup shredded mozzarella
- 1/4 cup grated Parmesan
- 1 teaspoon garlic powder
- Salt and pepper to taste
- Whole wheat pita, cut into triangles for dipping

Instructions:

1. Preheat the oven to 375°F (190°C).

2. In a bowl, mix together spinach, artichoke hearts, Greek yogurt, mayonnaise, mozzarella, Parmesan, garlic powder, salt, and pepper.

3. Transfer the mixture to a baking dish and bake for 25-30 minutes until bubbly and golden.

4. Serve with whole wheat pita for a satisfying and savory dip.

Nutrition Information (per serving):

- Calories: 150
- Protein: 8g
- Carbohydrates: 10g
- Fat: 9g
- Fiber: 3g
- Sugar: 2g
- Portion size: 1/4 cup dip with pita triangles

Chapter 6: Desserts

Embark on a sweet journey with these delectable dessert recipes designed for those with a sweet tooth and a mindful approach to managing diabetes. So, let's dive into the delightful world of diabetic-friendly desserts.

Berry and Yogurt Popsicles

Ingredients:

- 1 cup mixed berries (strawberries, blueberries, raspberries)
- 1 cup Greek yogurt (unsweetened)
- 2 tablespoons honey
- 1 teaspoon vanilla extract

Instructions:

1. In a blender, combine berries, Greek yogurt, honey, and vanilla extract.
2. Blend until smooth.
3. Pour the mixture into popsicle molds.
4. Freeze for at least 4 hours.

5. Enjoy these refreshing popsicles guilt-free!

Nutrition Information (per serving):

- Calories: 80
- Protein: 4g
- Carbohydrates: 15g
- Fat: 1g
- Fiber: 2g
- Sugar: 10g
- Portion Size: 1 popsicle

Dark Chocolate-Dipped Strawberries

Ingredients:

- 1 cup fresh strawberries
- 3 oz dark chocolate (70% cocoa or higher)

Instructions:

1. Melt dark chocolate in a microwave-safe bowl.
2. Dip each strawberry into the melted chocolate.
3. Place on a parchment-lined tray and let it cool.
4. Enjoy this simple yet elegant treat!

Nutrition Information (per serving):

- Calories: 60
- Protein: 1g
- Carbohydrates: 12g
- Fat: 3g
- Fiber: 3g
- Sugar: 7g
- Portion Size: 4 strawberries

Baked Apple with Cinnamon

Ingredients:

- 2 apples (cored and sliced)
- 1 teaspoon cinnamon
- 1 tablespoon lemon juice
- 1 tablespoon chopped nuts (optional)

Instructions:

1. Preheat oven to 350°F (175°C).
2. Toss apple slices with lemon juice and cinnamon.
3. Place in a baking dish and bake for 20-25 minutes.
4. Sprinkle with nuts before serving.

Nutrition Information (per serving):

- Calories: 90
- Protein: 1g
- Carbohydrates: 25g
- Fat: 0.5g
- Fiber: 5g
- Sugar: 18g
- Portion Size: 1/2 apple

Greek Yogurt and Honey Frozen Bites

Ingredients:

- 1 cup Greek yogurt (unsweetened)
- 2 tablespoons honey
- 1 teaspoon vanilla extract

Instructions:

1. Mix Greek yogurt, honey, and vanilla extract.
2. Spoon into ice cube trays.
3. Freeze for 2 hours.
4. Enjoy these bite-sized frozen delights!

Nutrition Information (per serving):

- Calories: 60
- Protein: 4g
- Carbohydrates: 10g
- Fat: 1.5g
- Fiber: 0g
- Sugar: 9g
- Portion Size: 4 bites

Sugar-Free Chocolate Avocado Mousse

Ingredients:

- 2 ripe avocados
- 1/4 cup unsweetened cocoa powder
- 1/4 cup almond milk (unsweetened)
- 1/4 cup sugar substitute (Stevia or Erythritol)
- 1 teaspoon vanilla extract

Instructions:

1. Blend avocados, cocoa powder, almond milk, sugar substitute, and vanilla extract until smooth.

2. Refrigerate for at least 1 hour.

3. Indulge in this rich and creamy chocolate mousse guilt-free!

Nutrition Information (per serving):

- Calories: 120

- Protein: 2g

- Carbohydrates: 10g

- Fat: 9g

- Fiber: 5g

- Sugar: 1g

- Portion Size: 1/2 cup

Almond Flour Banana Bread

Ingredients:

- 2 ripe bananas (mashed)

- 2 cups almond flour

- 3 eggs

- 1/4 cup coconut oil (melted)

- 1 teaspoon baking soda

- 1 teaspoon vanilla extract

- 1/2 teaspoon cinnamon

Instructions:

1. Preheat oven to 350°F (175°C).
2. Mix mashed bananas, almond flour, eggs, melted coconut oil, baking soda, vanilla extract, and cinnamon.
3. Pour into a greased loaf pan and bake for 30-35 minutes.
4. Slice and savor this moist and nutty banana bread!

Nutrition Information (per serving):

- Calories: 180
- Protein: 6g
- Carbohydrates: 12g
- Fat: 14g
- Fiber: 3g
- Sugar: 4g
- Portion Size: 1 slice

Lemon Sorbet with Fresh Mint

Ingredients:

- 3 cups water
- 1 cup lemon juice (freshly squeezed)

- 1/2 cup sugar substitute (Stevia or Erythritol)
- Fresh mint leaves (for garnish)

Instructions:

1. Mix water, lemon juice, and sugar substitute.
2. Pour into an ice cream maker and churn according to the manufacturer's instructions.
3. Garnish with fresh mint before serving.

Nutrition Information (per serving):

- Calories: 30
- Protein: 0g
- Carbohydrates: 8g
- Fat: 0g
- Fiber: 0g
- Sugar: 1g
- Portion Size: 1/2 cup

Pumpkin Pie Chia Pudding

Ingredients:

- 1/4 cup chia seeds
- 1 cup unsweetened almond milk

- 1/2 cup canned pumpkin puree
- 2 tablespoons maple syrup
- 1/2 teaspoon pumpkin pie spice

Instructions:

1. Mix chia seeds, almond milk, pumpkin puree, maple syrup, and pumpkin pie spice.
2. Refrigerate for at least 2 hours or overnight.
3. Enjoy this nutritious and flavorful chia pudding!

Nutrition Information (per serving):

- Calories: 90
- Protein: 3g
- Carbohydrates: 15g
- Fat: 3g
- Fiber: 7g
- Sugar: 5g
- Portion Size: 1/2 cup

Coconut and Berry Parfait

Ingredients:

- 1 cup mixed berries (strawberries, blueberries, raspberries)
- 1 cup coconut yogurt (unsweetened)
- 1/4 cup granola (sugar-free)

Instructions:

1. Layer coconut yogurt, mixed berries, and granola in a glass.
2. Repeat layers.
3. Top with a few berries for garnish.

Nutrition Information (per serving):

- Calories: 120
- Protein: 3g
- Carbohydrates: 18g
- Fat: 5g
- Fiber: 5g
- Sugar: 6g
- Portion Size: 1 cup

Walnut and Date Energy Bites

Ingredients:

- 1 cup walnuts
- 1 cup dates (pitted)
- 1/4 cup unsweetened cocoa powder
- 1 teaspoon vanilla extract
- Pinch of salt

Instructions:

1. Blend walnuts, dates, cocoa powder, vanilla extract, and salt until mixture sticks together.
2. Roll into bite-sized balls.
3. Refrigerate before serving.

Nutrition Information (per serving):

- Calories: 100
- Protein: 2g
- Carbohydrates: 12g
- Fat: 6g
- Fiber: 2g
- Sugar: 8g
- Portion Size: 2 bites

Raspberry and Almond Tart

Ingredients:

- 1 cup almond flour
- 2 tablespoons coconut oil (melted)
- 1/4 cup sugar substitute (Stevia or Erythritol)
- 1 cup fresh raspberries

Instructions:

1. Mix almond flour, melted coconut oil, and sugar substitute.
2. Press into a tart pan to form the crust.
3. Fill with fresh raspberries.
4. Chill before serving.

Nutrition Information (per serving):

- Calories: 150
- Protein: 3g
- Carbohydrates: 12g
- Fat: 11g
- Fiber: 5g
- Sugar: 2g
- Portion Size: 1/6 of the tart

Chia Seed and Mixed Berry Jam

Ingredients:

- 2 cups mixed berries (strawberries, blueberries, raspberries)
- 2 tablespoons chia seeds
- 1/4 cup sugar substitute (Stevia or Erythritol)

Instructions:

1. Mash berries and mix with chia seeds and sugar substitute.
2. Refrigerate until thickened.
3. Spread on toast or use as a topping.

Nutrition Information (per serving):

- Calories: 40
- Protein: 1g
- Carbohydrates: 9g
- Fat: 2g
- Fiber: 4g
- Sugar: 3g
- Portion Size: 2 tablespoons

Chocolate Zucchini Brownies

Ingredients:

- 2 cups shredded zucchini
- 1/2 cup almond flour
- 1/4 cup cocoa powder
- 1/4 cup sugar substitute (Stevia or Erythritol)
- 2 eggs
- 1 teaspoon vanilla extract

Instructions:

1. Preheat oven to 350°F (175°C).
2. Mix shredded zucchini, almond flour, cocoa powder, sugar substitute, eggs, and vanilla extract.
3. Pour into a greased baking pan and bake for 25-30 minutes.
4. Allow to cool before cutting into squares.

Nutrition Information (per serving):

- Calories: 80
- Protein: 3g
- Carbohydrates: 8g
- Fat: 5g

- Fiber: 2g

- Sugar: 3g

- Portion Size: 1 square

Mango and Coconut Frozen Yogurt

Ingredients:

- 1 cup frozen mango chunks

- 1 cup coconut yogurt (unsweetened)

- 2 tablespoons honey

Instructions:

1. Blend frozen mango, coconut yogurt, and honey until smooth.

2. Freeze for at least 2 hours.

3. Scoop and enjoy this tropical frozen delight!

Nutrition Information (per serving):

- Calories: 100

- Protein: 2g

- Carbohydrates: 18g

- Fat: 3g

- Fiber: 2g

- Sugar: 14g
- Portion Size: 1/2 cup

Peanut Butter and Banana Ice Cream

Ingredients:

- 2 ripe bananas (sliced and frozen)
- 2 tablespoons peanut butter
- 1/4 cup almond milk (unsweetened)

Instructions:

1. Blend frozen banana slices, peanut butter, and almond milk until creamy.
2. Freeze for an additional hour for a firmer texture.
3. Serve and relish this guilt-free ice cream!

Nutrition Information (per serving):

- Calories: 120
- Protein: 3g
- Carbohydrates: 20g
- Fat: 5g

- Fiber: 3g
- Sugar: 10g
- Portion Size: 1/2 cup

Chapter 7: Smoothies

In this chapter, we present a vibrant collection of smoothie recipes that not only tantalize your taste buds but also pack a nutritional punch. Let's dive into the world of vibrant colors, enticing flavors, and nourishing ingredients.

Green Power Smoothie with Kale and Pineapple

Ingredients:

- 1 cup kale leaves, stemmed
- 1/2 cup pineapple chunks
- 1 banana
- 1/2 cup Greek yogurt
- 1 tablespoon chia seeds
- 1 cup water or coconut water

Instructions:

1. Combine kale, pineapple, banana, Greek yogurt, chia seeds, and water in a blender.
2. Blend until smooth.

3. Pour into a glass and enjoy!

Nutrition Information:

- Calories: 180
- Protein: 8g
- Carbohydrates: 30g
- Fat: 4g
- Fiber: 7g
- Sugar: 15g
- Portion Size: 1 serving

Berry Blast Smoothie with Greek Yogurt

Ingredients:

- 1 cup mixed berries (strawberries, blueberries, raspberries)
- 1/2 cup Greek yogurt
- 1 tablespoon honey
- 1/2 cup almond milk
- Ice cubes (optional)

Instructions:

1. Blend mixed berries, Greek yogurt, honey, and almond milk until smooth.

2. Add ice cubes if desired and blend again.

3. Pour into a glass and savor the berry goodness!

Nutrition Information:

- Calories: 160

- Protein: 7g

- Carbohydrates: 25g

- Fat: 3g

- Fiber: 5g

- Sugar: 18g

- Portion Size: 1 serving

Avocado and Spinach Smoothie

Ingredients:

- 1/2 avocado

- 1 cup spinach leaves

- 1/2 banana

- 1/2 cup plain yogurt

- 1 tablespoon flaxseeds

- 1 cup water or almond milk

Instructions:

1. Blend avocado, spinach, banana, yogurt, flaxseeds, and water (or almond milk) until creamy.
2. Pour into a glass and enjoy the nourishing goodness!

Nutrition Information:

- Calories: 220
- Protein: 6g
- Carbohydrates: 18g
- Fat: 15g
- Fiber: 7g
- Sugar: 6g
- Portion Size: 1 serving

Mango and Coconut Water Smoothie

Ingredients:

- 1 cup ripe mango, diced
- 1/2 cup coconut water
- 1/2 cup plain Greek yogurt
- 1 tablespoon hemp seeds

- Ice cubes (optional)

Instructions:

1. Blend mango, coconut water, Greek yogurt, and hemp seeds until smooth.
2. Add ice cubes if desired and blend again.
3. Pour into a glass and transport yourself to a tropical paradise!

Nutrition Information:

- Calories: 200
- Protein: 9g
- Carbohydrates: 30g
- Fat: 6g
- Fiber: 5g
- Sugar: 20g
- Portion Size: 1 serving

Chocolate Peanut Butter Protein Smoothie

Ingredients:

- 1 scoop chocolate protein powder
- 2 tablespoons peanut butter
- 1 banana
- 1 cup unsweetened almond milk
- Ice cubes (optional)

Instructions:

1. Blend chocolate protein powder, peanut butter, banana, and almond milk until well combined.
2. Add ice cubes if desired and blend again.
3. Pour into a glass and indulge in this protein-packed delight!

Nutrition Information:

- Calories: 280
- Protein: 25g
- Carbohydrates: 22g
- Fat: 12g
- Fiber: 6g

- Sugar: 10g

- Portion Size: 1 serving

Tropical Paradise Smoothie with Mango and Kiwi

Ingredients:

- 1/2 cup diced mango

- 1 kiwi, peeled and sliced

- 1/2 cup pineapple juice

- 1/2 cup coconut milk

- 1 tablespoon chia seeds

Instructions:

1. Blend mango, kiwi, pineapple juice, coconut milk, and chia seeds until smooth.

2. Pour into a glass and feel the tropical vibes!

Nutrition Information:

- Calories: 220

- Protein: 5g

- Carbohydrates: 30g

- Fat: 10g
- Fiber: 8g
- Sugar: 18g
- Portion Size: 1 serving

Blueberry and Almond Milk Smoothie

Ingredients:

- 1 cup blueberries (fresh or frozen)
- 1/2 cup almond milk
- 1/2 cup plain yogurt
- 1 tablespoon almond butter
- 1 teaspoon honey

Instructions:

1. Blend blueberries, almond milk, yogurt, almond butter, and honey until smooth.
2. Pour into a glass and relish the antioxidant-rich goodness!

Nutrition Information:

- Calories: 180
- Protein: 8g
- Carbohydrates: 25g
- Fat: 7g
- Fiber: 6g
- Sugar: 15g
- Portion Size: 1 serving

Coffee and Banana Protein Smoothie

Ingredients:

- 1/2 cup cold brewed coffee
- 1 banana
- 1 scoop vanilla protein powder
- 1/2 cup unsweetened almond milk
- Ice cubes (optional)

Instructions:

1. Blend cold brewed coffee, banana, protein powder, and almond milk until creamy.

2. Add ice cubes if desired and blend again.

3. Pour into a glass and enjoy a caffeinated protein boost!

Nutrition Information:

- Calories: 210
- Protein: 20g
- Carbohydrates: 26g
- Fat: 4g
- Fiber: 5g
- Sugar: 12g
- Portion Size: 1 serving

Spinach and Pineapple Smoothie

Ingredients:

- 1 cup fresh spinach leaves
- 1/2 cup pineapple chunks
- 1/2 banana
- 1/2 cup coconut water
- 1 tablespoon flaxseeds

Instructions:

1. Blend spinach, pineapple, banana, coconut water, and flaxseeds until smooth.

2. Pour into a glass and savor the refreshing taste of greens!

Nutrition Information:

- Calories: 160
- Protein: 6g
- Carbohydrates: 30g
- Fat: 4g
- Fiber: 7g
- Sugar: 15g
- Portion Size: 1 serving

Strawberry and Chia Seed Smoothie

Ingredients:

- 1 cup fresh strawberries, hulled
- 1/2 cup plain Greek yogurt
- 1 tablespoon chia seeds
- 1/2 cup almond milk
- Ice cubes (optional)

Instructions:

1. Blend strawberries, Greek yogurt, chia seeds, and almond milk until smooth.
2. Add ice cubes if desired and blend again.
3. Pour into a glass and enjoy the luscious sweetness of strawberries!

Nutrition Information:

- Calories: 170
- Protein: 8g
- Carbohydrates: 22g
- Fat: 6g
- Fiber: 7g
- Sugar: 12g
- Portion Size: 1 serving

Peach and Greek Yogurt Smoothie

Ingredients:

- 1 ripe peach, pitted and sliced
- 1/2 cup plain Greek yogurt
- 1/2 cup orange juice
- 1 tablespoon honey

- 1/2 teaspoon vanilla extract

Instructions:

1. Blend peach, Greek yogurt, orange juice, honey, and vanilla extract until well combined.
2. Pour into a glass and revel in the peachy goodness!

Nutrition Information:

- Calories: 200
- Protein: 9g
- Carbohydrates: 28g
- Fat: 5g
- Fiber: 4g
- Sugar: 22g
- Portion Size: 1 serving

Cucumber and Mint Green Smoothie

Ingredients:

- 1/2 cucumber, peeled and sliced
- 1 cup fresh spinach leaves
- 1/4 cup fresh mint leaves
- 1/2 green apple, cored and chopped

- 1/2 cup coconut water

Instructions:

1. Blend cucumber, spinach, mint, green apple, and coconut water until smooth.
2. Pour into a glass and enjoy the cool and refreshing taste!

Nutrition Information:

- Calories: 140
- Protein: 4g
- Carbohydrates: 30g
- Fat: 2g
- Fiber: 6g
- Sugar: 18g
- Portion Size: 1 serving

Watermelon and Lime Refresher

Ingredients:

- 1 cup fresh watermelon, diced
- Juice of 1 lime
- 1/2 cup coconut water

- 1 tablespoon chia seeds
- Ice cubes (optional)

Instructions:

1. Blend watermelon, lime juice, coconut water, and chia seeds until refreshing and smooth.
2. Add ice cubes if desired and blend again.
3. Pour into a glass and experience the hydrating bliss of watermelon!

Nutrition Information:

- Calories: 120
- Protein: 3g
- Carbohydrates: 25g
- Fat: 2g
- Fiber: 5g
- Sugar: 18g
- Portion Size: 1 serving

Orange Creamsicle Smoothie

Ingredients:

- 1 orange, peeled and segmented

- 1/2 cup plain Greek yogurt
- 1/2 cup almond milk
- 1 tablespoon honey
- 1/2 teaspoon vanilla extract

Instructions:

1. Blend orange segments, Greek yogurt, almond milk, honey, and vanilla extract until creamy.
2. Pour into a glass and relish the nostalgic flavor of an orange creamsicle!

Nutrition Information:

- Calories: 180
- Protein: 7g
- Carbohydrates: 30g
- Fat: 4g
- Fiber: 5g
- Sugar: 20g
- Portion Size: 1 serving

Mixed Berry and Oat Smoothie

Ingredients:

- 1 cup mixed berries (strawberries, blueberries, raspberries)
- 1/2 cup rolled oats
- 1/2 cup plain Greek yogurt
- 1 tablespoon almond butter
- 1 cup almond milk

Instructions:

1. Blend mixed berries, rolled oats, Greek yogurt, almond butter, and almond milk until smooth.
2. Pour into a glass and enjoy the delightful combination of berries and oats!

Nutrition Information:

- Calories: 230
- Protein: 10g
- Carbohydrates: 30g
- Fat: 9g
- Fiber: 7g
- Sugar: 12g
- Portion Size: 1 serving

CONCLUSION

As we close the chapters of this book, we hope to leave you not only with a diverse array of delicious recipes but also with a newfound sense of empowerment. Managing diabetes doesn't have to mean sacrificing taste or culinary enjoyment. Instead, it becomes an opportunity to explore the rich tapestry of flavors that nourish both the body and the soul.

The 30-day meal plan serves as a structured foundation, guiding you through a month of balanced, satisfying, and diabetic-friendly meals. From the wholesome breakfasts that kickstart your day to the savory dinners that bring it to a close, each recipe is crafted with your health and taste buds in mind.

Whether it's the vibrant salads, the comforting soups, or the delectable desserts, every dish is a testament to the idea that eating well can be a joyous experience. The snacks and appetizers add a delightful touch to your daily routine, proving that even moments of indulgence can align with your dietary goals.

Desserts, often seen as off-limits, become a celebration of natural sweetness and innovative combinations. And the refreshing smoothies not only offer a burst of energy but also elevate the concept of a beverage to a nutrient-packed, enjoyable treat.

In the world of diabetes management, knowledge is power. The insights provided in the introduction lay the foundation for understanding the crucial relationship between diet and diabetes. Armed with this knowledge, you're equipped to make informed choices that positively impact your well-being.

As you navigate the pages of this cookbook, we encourage you to embrace the diversity of ingredients, experiment with flavors, and make these recipes your own. The journey to wellness is not just about what you eat but how you savor each bite, creating a mindful connection between food and body.

Remember, this cookbook is not a rigid set of rules but a flexible guide designed to inspire and support you on your diabetic journey. Embrace the joy of cooking, relish the vibrant flavors, and celebrate the fact that, with every meal, you're nurturing both your body and your spirit.

May this cookbook be a trusted companion, empowering you to not only manage diabetes but to thrive, savoring the richness of a life well-lived. Here's to your health, happiness, and the delicious possibilities that lie ahead.